NUTRITION ESSENTIALS

A COMPREHENSIVE GUIDE TO HEALTHFUL

EATING

CYRIL LAKES

Contents

CHAPTER ONE

INTRODUCTION

In a world full of trendy superfoods, contradicting nutrition advice, and fad diets, learning and practicing the art of healthful eating may be an intimidating and stressful task. In the middle of the chaos and uncertainty, finding the right nutrition becomes more than just knowing what to eat it also involves figuring out how to make sense of the abundance of information accessible and navigating the complexity of today's food scene.

Welcome to "Nutrition Essentials: A Comprehensive Guide to Healthful Eating." This book is a roadmap to help you navigate the complex world of nutrition with clarity, confidence, and empowerment. It's not simply another diet plan or fast fix. This guide is intended to give you the information, resources, and techniques you need to make wise decisions and succeed in your nutritional journey— whether your goal is to manage a particular health issue, enhance your general well-being, or simply develop a more harmonious and fulfilling relationship with food.

We'll go deeply into the fundamentals of nutrition in this extensive book, covering the elements of a healthy diet, comprehending the science behind food and its effects on our bodies, and identifying the critical elements that support general wellbeing. Every chapter in this book from macronutrients to micronutrients, from dietary patterns to mindful eating practices has been painstakingly designed to give you useful advice, evidence-based suggestions, and doable actions to help you maximize the potential of nutrition for your health and vitality.

However, "Nutrition Essentials" offers a comprehensive strategy for fueling your body, mind, and spirit it's not just a collection of statistics and facts. We'll look at how nutrition relates to other aspects of wellness, like exercise, mental health, and lifestyle decisions, to provide a whole picture of what it really means to be healthy and successful in today's hectic world.

You will gain the ability to take back control of your relationship with food, develop a better awareness of the special requirements of your body, and adopt a sustainable, pleasurable, and rewarding lifestyle of eating healthily. "Nutrition Essentials" is your reliable travel companion on the road to greater health and energy, regardless of your level of experience or familiarity with nutritional wellness.

So come along with me as we go out on this life-changing adventure toward a nutritious diet. Let's investigate the fundamentals of nutrition, discover how to fuel our bodies from the inside out, and set out on a lifetime journey toward the best possible health, vigor, and well-being.

The Basics of Nutrition

A. The macronutrients fats, proteins, and carbohydrates

The basic dietary components known as macronutrients give us energy and support a number of biological processes. Maintaining a balanced diet requires an understanding of their responsibilities and sources:

The body uses carbohydrates as its main energy source to power both bodily processes and mental processes. Foods like grains, fruits, vegetables, and legumes contain them. Despite being demonized in some diet fads, carbohydrates are an essential component of a balanced diet because they provide fiber, vitamins, and minerals.

Proteins: Building and mending tissues, bolstering immunological response, and generating hormones and enzymes all depend on proteins. Meat, poultry, fish, eggs, dairy products, legumes, nuts, and seeds are dietary sources of protein. To guarantee that you are getting enough of the essential amino acids, it is crucial to eat a range of protein sources.

Fats: Rich in energy, fats are essential for the synthesis of hormones, the construction of cells, and the absorption of nutrients. Nuts, seeds, avocados, olive oil, and fatty fish are good sources of healthy fats that are good for your heart and general health. Reducing the amount of saturated and trans fats consumed from fried and processed meals is crucial in lowering the risk of developing chronic illnesses.

B. Minerals and vitamins are micronutrients.

Essential nutrients known as micronutrients are needed in trace levels for a variety of physiological processes. They are essential for immunological response, metabolism, and general health:

Vitamins: Vitamins are organic substances that are essential for growth, development, and the prevention of disease. They also function as cofactors in enzyme reactions. They are divided into two groups: fat-soluble vitamins (such vitamins A, D, E, and K) and water-soluble vitamins (like vitamin C and the B vitamins). Getting enough vitamins requires eating a wide variety of fruits, vegetables, whole grains, and other nutrient-dense foods.

Minerals are inorganic substances that are necessary for the proper functioning of nerves, bones, fluid equilibrium, and other physiological systems. While trace elements like iron, zinc, selenium, and copper are needed in lower amounts, major minerals like calcium, magnesium, sodium, and potassium are needed in larger proportions. A varied diet rich in fruits, vegetables, whole grains, lean meats, dairy products, and other nutrients can help guarantee that the body gets enough minerals.

C. The Value of Hydration and Water

Although it is frequently disregarded, water is possibly the most important ingredient for survival and general wellness. It is essential for maintaining digestion, lubricating joints, carrying nutrients and waste materials, and controlling body temperature. sustaining proper hydration is crucial for sustaining mental clarity, physical stamina, and general health.

It's essential to maintain adequate hydration for both performance and wellness. To make sure you're well hydrated, try to drink water throughout the day and be aware of thirst signals. To increase overall fluid consumption, hydrating meals including fruits, vegetables, soups, and smoothies can be consumed in addition to water.

Dietary guidelines are evidence-based suggestions created by medical authorities to encourage a healthy diet and lower the chance of developing chronic illnesses. These recommendations provide a framework within which people, families, and communities can make educated food decisions. The following are some essential dietary guidelines to comprehend:

Basis in Scientific Research: To reflect the most recent findings on nutrition and health, dietary guidelines are periodically updated and based on scientific research. Expert panels or advisory committees made up of medical professionals, nutrition scientists, and other subject matter experts create them.

Emphasis on Food categories and Nutrients: Eating a range of nutrient-dense foods from all food categories is recommended by most dietary guidelines. Based on age, sex, and other personal characteristics, they offer dietary recommendations for the consumption of macronutrients (proteins, carbs, and fats) and micronutrients (vitamins and minerals).

Dietary guidelines provide a strong emphasis on moderation and balance in eating choices, stressing the need of eating a variety of foods in sensible amounts. They advise reducing consumption of foods and nutrients such added sugars, saturated fats, and sodium that may aggravate chronic illnesses.

Encouragement of Healthful Eating Patterns: Fruits, vegetables, whole grains, lean meats, and healthy fats are all part of a diet rich in recommended daily allowances. They stress the value of eating a range of meals rich in nutrients and minimizing the use of ultra-processed and processed foods, sugar-filled drinks, and foods high in sodium and saturated fats.

Adaptability to Dietary and Cultural Preferences: Dietary recommendations are made to accommodate a wide range of dietary and cultural preferences. They acknowledge that there is no one-size-fits-all approach to nutrition and advise people to tailor their diets according to their cultural customs, individual tastes, and health objectives.

Practical Advice for Everyday Living: Dietary guidelines offer helpful advice for incorporating nutrition science into regular meal planning and food selections. They frequently contain advice on how to shop for groceries, prepare meals, eat out, and make healthier decisions in a variety of situations.

All things considered, knowing dietary recommendations is critical to make wise choices about food and nourishment. People can lower their long-term risk of developing chronic diseases and enhance their general health and well-being by implementing healthy eating habits and adhering to evidence-based recommendations.

Nutrition's Function in Health

A. Dietary Approaches to Prevent Chronic Diseases:

The prevention of chronic diseases is one of nutrition's most important contributions to general health. A nutritious diet has been repeatedly linked to a lower chance of acquiring heart disease, diabetes, hypertension, obesity, and some types of cancer, among other chronic illnesses. People can provide their bodies vital nutrients and antioxidants that promote general health and lower inflammation by eating a diet high in fruits, vegetables, whole grains, lean meats, and healthy fats. Limiting processed meals, sugar-filled drinks, and foods heavy in sodium and saturated fats can also help prolong life and reduce the risk of chronic illnesses.

B. Increasing Immune Function with Foods High in Nutrients:

In order to maintain immune system function and protect the body from infections and illnesses, nutrition is essential. A number of nutrients, including zinc, vitamins A, C, D, and E, are necessary for the immune system to operate properly. A diet high in fruits, vegetables, nuts, seeds, and lean meats can supply the body with the antioxidants, vitamins, and minerals it needs to maintain a healthy immune system. Furthermore, consuming fiber-rich foods and probiotics can help maintain a healthy gut microbiome and stay hydrated, both of which can improve immune function and lower the risk of infection.

C. Improving Cognitive and Mental Health:

Mental well-being and cognitive performance are also significantly impacted by nutrition. Studies have indicated that specific nutrients, including antioxidants, B vitamins, and omega-3 fatty acids, are critical for neurotransmitter activity and overall brain health. Along with other healthful foods, eating a diet high in these nutrients can help regulate mood, lower the risk of anxiety and depression, and improve memory and cognitive function.

CHAPTER TWO

Furthermore, there is a correlation between the adoption of nutritious eating habits, like the Mediterranean diet or the DASH (Dietary Approaches to Stop Hypertension) diet, and a decreased risk of cognitive decline and neurodegenerative disorders, such dementia and Alzheimer's disease.

All things considered, diet has a variety of effects on immune system function, chronic illness prevention, mental and cognitive performance, and overall health and well-being. People may maximize their nutrition and support their bodies' innate ability to thrive by making nutrient-rich foods a priority and developing healthy eating habits.

Assembling an Equilibrium Plate

A. The Value of a Diverse Diet

A diet rich in nutrients and well-balanced must be varied. Eating a variety of foods guarantees that you will receive a broad spectrum of antioxidants, vitamins, minerals, and nutrients that promote general health and wellbeing. When preparing meals and snacks, try to incorporate items from all the food groups, such as whole grains, fruits, vegetables, lean meats, and healthy fats. Try a variety of flavors, textures, and cooking techniques to keep your meals interesting and fulfilling. You may maximize your nutrient intake and reap a wider range of health benefits by embracing variety in your diet.

B. Making Well-Balanced Snacks and Meals:

A combination of macronutrients (proteins, fats, and carbs) and micronutrients (vitamins and minerals) found in balanced meals and snacks improve satiety, energy levels, and general health. Aim to incorporate a variety of nutrient-rich items from each food group while assembling a balanced plate:

Fruits and Vegetables: These vibrant, high-fiber, high-mineral, high-antioxidant foods should make up half of your plate. To optimize your intake of nutrients, select a range of fruit with varying hues and textures.

Whole Grains: To get fiber, vitamins, minerals, and long-lasting energy, include whole grains in your meals. Examples of these are brown rice, quinoa, oats, and whole wheat bread, pasta, and cereals.

Lean Proteins: To promote muscular health, satiety, and general nutrition, include lean protein sources in your meals, such as chicken, fish, tofu, beans, lentils, and low-fat dairy products.

Healthy Fats: To promote heart health, cognitive function, and nutrient absorption, include sources of healthy fats in your meals, such as avocados, nuts, seeds, olive oil, and fatty fish.

Dairy or Dairy substitutes: If you're looking for calcium, vitamin D, and protein, go for dairy or fortified dairy substitutes like milk, yogurt, and cheese.

To stay full and energized in between meals, try to incorporate a mix of carbohydrates, proteins, and fats in your snack plans. Try pairing whole grain crackers with cheese, Greek yogurt with berries, or apple slices with peanut butter.

C. Mindful Eating and Portion Control:

To create a balanced plate and keep a positive connection with food, portion control and mindful eating are critical. To prevent overeating and aid in weight management, pay attention to serving and portion sizes. To determine the right portion sizes for various food groups, use visual clues like the size of a deck of cards or your hand.

Eat mindfully by taking your time, enjoying every bite, and being aware of your body's signals of hunger and fullness. When dining, stay away from distractions like television or electronics and concentrate on the flavors and textures of the food. Pay attention to your body's signals of hunger and fullness, and stop eating when you're satisfied but not too full.

You may create a balanced plate that supports general health, energy levels, and well-being by emphasizing variety, preparing balanced meals and snacks, exercising portion control, and engaging in mindful eating.

Eating Well Throughout Life

A. Infant and Toddler Nutrition:

The formative years are crucial for a child's growth, development, and the establishment of a good diet. Breast milk or formula gives babies (0–12 months old) the nutrition they need for healthy growth and development. Around six months of age, solid food should be introduced while breastfeeding or using formula to help expose babies to a range of flavors and textures. Offering a balanced diet with a range of nutrient-rich foods, such as fruits, vegetables, whole grains, lean proteins, and healthy fats, is crucial as babies grow into toddlers (1-3 years old). Positive eating habits and independence are facilitated by age-appropriate portion sizes and encouragement of self-feeding.

B. Nutrition in Childhood and Good Eating Practices:

Childhood is a crucial time for forming food habits that last a lifetime and for fostering the best possible growth and development. To ensure that children get all the nutrients they need, it is crucial to encourage them to consume a balanced diet that consists of a range of foods from all food groups. Limit the consumption of processed foods, sugary snacks, and sweetened beverages and emphasize the value of fruits, vegetables, whole grains, lean proteins, and healthy fats. To encourage healthy eating habits and positive attitudes about food, plan and prepare meals as a family and involve the kids. Teach kids the value of following their hunger and fullness cues and making nutrient-dense decisions.

C. Adolescent and Young Adult Nutrition:

There is a lot of growth and development during adolescence and early adulthood, along with nutritional and lifestyle changes. Adolescents and young adults should eat a balanced diet that gives them the energy and nutrients they need to maintain their overall health, scholastic success, and physical growth. Urge teenagers and young people to prioritize eating regular meals and snacks, make healthy food choices, and drink enough of water. Insist that people eat breakfast, choose whole grains, lean proteins, and healthy fats, and include fruits and vegetables in their meals and snacks. Teach teenagers and young adults the importance of good nutrition for both physical and mental health, as well as how it can help prevent chronic illnesses and enhance overall wellbeing.

People can establish the groundwork for a lifetime of health and well-being by emphasizing nutrition throughout the lifespan and encouraging wholesome eating habits from early childhood through young adulthood. Families, schools, and communities should be encouraged to promote healthy eating habits. They should also be given the tools and information necessary to enable people to make nourishing decisions at every stage of life.

Part I: Interpreting Nutrition Labels

Nutrition labels give consumers important information on the nutritional makeup of packaged foods and drinks, enabling them to make educated diet decisions. Pay particular attention to these crucial elements while interpreting nutrition labels:

portion Size: All additional nutritional information is based on the portion size indicated at the top of the label, so pay close attention to it.

Calories: To determine how many calories you will get from the product, look at the quantity of calories per serving.

macronutrients: Verify the breakdown of saturated and trans fats, as well as the amounts of carbs, proteins, and fats in each meal.

Micronutrients: Examine the label's percentages of recommended daily intake for the vitamins and minerals that are considered important micronutrients.

components List: Look over the components list to be sure there are no artificial ingredients, preservatives, or additives.

B. Recognizing Added Ingredients and Hidden Sugars:

A lot of processed meals and drinks include extra ingredients and hidden sugars that can lead to overindulgence in calories and bad health consequences. When examining product labels, keep an eye out for the following sources of extra ingredients and hidden sugars:

Among the first few ingredients are several types of sugar, such as sucrose, maltose, dextrose, and high fructose corn syrup.

Products labeled as "sugar-free" or "diet" may contain artificial sweeteners and sugar alcohols (such as aspartame, saccharin, and sorbitol).

Trans fats and hydrogenated oils, which go by numerous names (such partially hydrogenated oils), raise the risk of heart disease.

Preservatives, artificial colors, and tastes are added to improve shelf life, taste, and appearance.

C. Getting Around Food Advertising and Marketing:

Food choices, purchase patterns, and customer preferences are greatly influenced by food marketing and promotion. To help you make wise selections when navigating food marketing and advertising, take into account the following strategies:

Be wary of marketing slogans and health claims that seem too good to be true.

For accurate information about the composition of a product, go past marketing and the label on the front of the packaging to the nutrition label and ingredients list.

Examine the context of marketing communications to see if they support dietary guidelines and healthy eating habits.

By talking about the strategies utilized in food marketing and advertising and encouraging media literacy skills, you can teach kids and teenagers how to be discriminating consumers.

Consumers may prioritize healthy eating habits and make better educated diet decisions by learning how to read nutrition labels, spot additional ingredients and hidden sugars, and manage food marketing and advertising. Urge people to actively participate in the process of reading food labels, challenging marketing messaging, and fighting for clear and truthful food information.

CHAPTER THREE

Food and Emotional Well-Being

A. Gut-Brain Flow and Psychological Health:

The complex interaction known as the gut-brain axis between the gut and the brain has been clarified by recent studies. Trillions of microbes reside in the gut and are essential for immunological response, digestion, and even mood management. This intricate web of fungus, bacteria, and other microbes influences mood, emotional health, and cognitive function by producing neurotransmitters and interacting with the brain via the vagus nerve. Better mental health outcomes are linked to a healthy gut microbiome, whereas dysbiosis (imbalance) may be a factor in diseases including stress, anxiety, and depression. Eating a diet high in fiber, fermented foods, probiotics, and prebiotics enhances gut health and may have a good effect on mental health.

B. Foods that Promote Mood and Mental Health:

Due to their provision of vital nutrients for brain function and neurotransmitter synthesis, several foods and nutrients have been demonstrated to promote mental health and mood. For instance, omega-3 fatty acids, which are essential for brain function and may lessen the symptoms of anxiety and depression, are found in walnuts, chia seeds, flaxseeds, and fatty fish. Antioxidant-rich foods include berries, dark leafy greens, and colorful fruits and vegetables. These foods also help fight inflammation and oxidative stress, which are connected to mood problems. Furthermore, the presence of complex carbs in whole grains, legumes, and starchy vegetables helps to maintain stable blood sugar levels and the generation of serotonin, which in turn promotes feelings of wellbeing and tranquility.

C. Nutritional Techniques for Managing Stress:

Prolonged stress can negatively impact mood, sleep, appetite, and cognitive function, as well as mental health and general wellbeing. When it comes to stress management and building resilience against its consequences, nutrition is crucial. During stressful times, maintaining a balanced diet that provides enough protein, complex carbs, healthy fats, and vitamins helps maintain energy levels and cognitive performance. Including foods that assist reduce stress, such avocados, almonds, seeds, fatty fish, leafy greens, and nuts, gives the nervous system support and helps control the body's stress response. Furthermore, mindful eating, drinking plenty of water, and placing a high value on self-care practices like regular exercise, learning relaxation techniques, and getting enough sleep all help with stress management and mental health.

People can take proactive measures to improve mental wellbeing and resilience in the face of life's challenges by being aware of the link between nutrition and mental health and using dietary choices that support brain health and emotional well-being. A comprehensive approach to mental health that nourishes the mind, body, and spirit includes including nutrient-rich foods, supporting a healthy gut microbiota, and placing a high value on self-care routines.

Handling Intolerances and Allergies to Food

A. Comprehending Food Sensitivities and Allergies:

Food allergies and intolerances are reactions caused by the immune system to particular meals or components. When a specific food protein is consumed, food allergies cause an immunological reaction that can result in symptoms including hives, swelling, breathing difficulties, and, in extreme situations, anaphylaxis. Peanuts, tree nuts, fish, shellfish, eggs, milk, soy, wheat, and sesame are examples of common food allergies. Contrarily, food intolerances cause digestive problems such bloating, gas, diarrhea, or abdominal pain because they inhibit particular enzymes or cause sensitivity to certain food ingredients. Common food intolerances include gluten intolerance (celiac illness or non-celiac gluten sensitivity) and lactose intolerance (inability to digest lactose in dairy products). It is essential to distinguish between food allergies and intolerances in order to make an accurate diagnosis and provide the right care.

B. Handling Dietary Limitations and Steering Clear of Triggers:

It's important to pay close attention to ingredient labels, food preparation techniques, and cross-contamination hazards when managing food allergies and intolerances. To avoid sometimes fatal responses, people with food allergies must abstain from consuming even trace amounts of their allergen. Essential strategies for preventing allergen exposure include asking questions about ingredients while dining out, reading food labels for allergen information, and alerting food service providers of dietary preferences. Finding and removing trigger items from the diet can help people with food intolerances feel better and have less discomfort in their gastrointestinal tract. A licensed dietician or healthcare professional can offer individualized advice on how to manage dietary restrictions and create safe, well-balanced meal plans.

C. Identifying Fun and Secure Substitutes:

Taste, diversity, and enjoyment of food are not sacrificed when one has dietary allergies or intolerances. Thankfully, those with dietary limitations have access to a wide variety of delicious and healthy substitutes. More and more food producers are producing allergy-friendly items, such as soy-free protein sources, nut-free snacks, gluten-free grains and flours, and dairy-free milk substitutes. People can still enjoy their favorite dishes while avoiding allergies or intolerances by experimenting with different components and recipes. Discovering the cuisines of other nations might also introduce you to new flavors and ingredients that work with your diet. People with food allergies and intolerances can manage their dietary limitations and have delicious, nutrient-dense meals if they are creative, adaptable, and receive support from medical professionals and community resources.

Through comprehension of food allergies and intolerances, use of dietary restriction management measures, and investigation of safe and pleasurable substitutes, people can sustain a nutritious and satisfying diet that meets their particular dietary requirements and enhances their general well-being.

Overcoming Obstacles to a Healthful Diet

A. Handling Food Cravings and Emotional Eating:

Maintaining a healthy diet can be seriously hampered by emotional eating and food cravings. Comfort foods that are heavy in sugar, fat, and calories can become craved in response to stress, boredom, sadness, and other emotions. Developing other coping strategies for handling emotions other than eating is crucial to overcoming emotional eating. Those who engage in activities like yoga, meditation, or journaling, or who practice mindfulness, deep breathing exercises, can become more conscious of their emotions and learn healthy coping mechanisms. Creating a network of friends, family, or a therapist to lean on can help provide extra accountability and support for controlling emotional eating habits.

B. Choosing Healthier Options When Eating Out:

Making healthy food choices when dining out or attending social events can be difficult because many menu items are heavy in calories, sodium, and bad fats. It's helpful to plan ahead when dining out by looking over menus online, selecting restaurants that serve healthier options, and steering clear of fast food and all-you-can-eat buffets. When placing your order, choose baked, steamed, or grilled foods over fried or breaded ones, and ask for dressings and sauces to be served on the side. Furthermore, divide entrees with a friend or request a to-go box to save half the meal for later to further practice portion control. Overeating when dining out can be avoided by paying attention to portion sizes and paying attention to signals of hunger and fullness.

C. Handling Food Environments and Social Pressures:

Eating habits can be influenced by social pressures and food environments, which can make it difficult to maintain healthy choices. Social pressure from peers, cultural customs, and food-focused get-togethers can encourage people to overindulge in unhealthy meals or serve larger portions. It's critical to discuss dietary preferences and goals with friends, family, and coworkers in order to manage social pressures and food environments. You should also ask for their assistance in making healthy decisions. To prevent overindulging in less nutrient-dense foods, bring a healthy dish to share or eat a small, balanced meal before attending social gatherings or events. Additionally, stock the kitchen with wholesome foods and reduce the amount of alluring, high-calorie snacks and treats to foster a supportive home environment.

Through the adoption of coping mechanisms for emotional eating, making nutritious decisions when dining out, and navigating social pressures and food environments, people can surmount common obstacles to eating a healthy diet and accomplish their nutrition objectives. Developing resilient habits, engaging in mindfulness exercises, and asking for support from others can assist people in creating enduring routines that promote general health and wellbeing.

Summary

To sum up, eating a healthy diet is a complex process that calls for consideration of a number of variables, such as dietary preferences, environmental influences, lifestyle choices, and nutritional requirements. We have covered the foundational ideas of nutrition, methods for choosing wholesome foods, and solutions for typical obstacles to eating well throughout this extensive guide. All facets of eating healthily contribute to general vitality and well-being, from realizing the value of balanced nutrition to navigating dietary restrictions and social pressures.

As we come to the end of this journey, it is important to stress that eating healthfully is about making decisions that support our mental, emotional, and physical well-being rather than about being perfect. It's about providing our bodies with nutrient-dense foods, developing a healthy relationship with food, and adopting a flexible and enjoyable balanced eating style. People can improve their longevity, lower their chance of developing chronic illnesses, and improve their quality of life by making healthy eating habits a priority.

Let us continue to practice self-awareness, resilience, and mindfulness in our food choices as we progress on our paths to health and wellness. Let us strive to nourish our bodies with wholesome foods, honor our individual needs and preferences, and find joy and satisfaction in the nourishing power of food. Together, let us embrace the path to healthful eating and embrace a future of vibrant health and well-being for ourselves and generations to come.

THE END